Beauty Secrets of Natural Skincare:

Including Acne Fighting Tips & Anti-Aging Tricks

Disclaimer:

This eBook was written by Inner Glow. We are not physicians and cannot be held liable for the information written here. It is not intended to provide medical advice. Please do not use it as an alternative to seeking help from a medical professional.

Table of Contents

Chapter 1 –
Going Natural

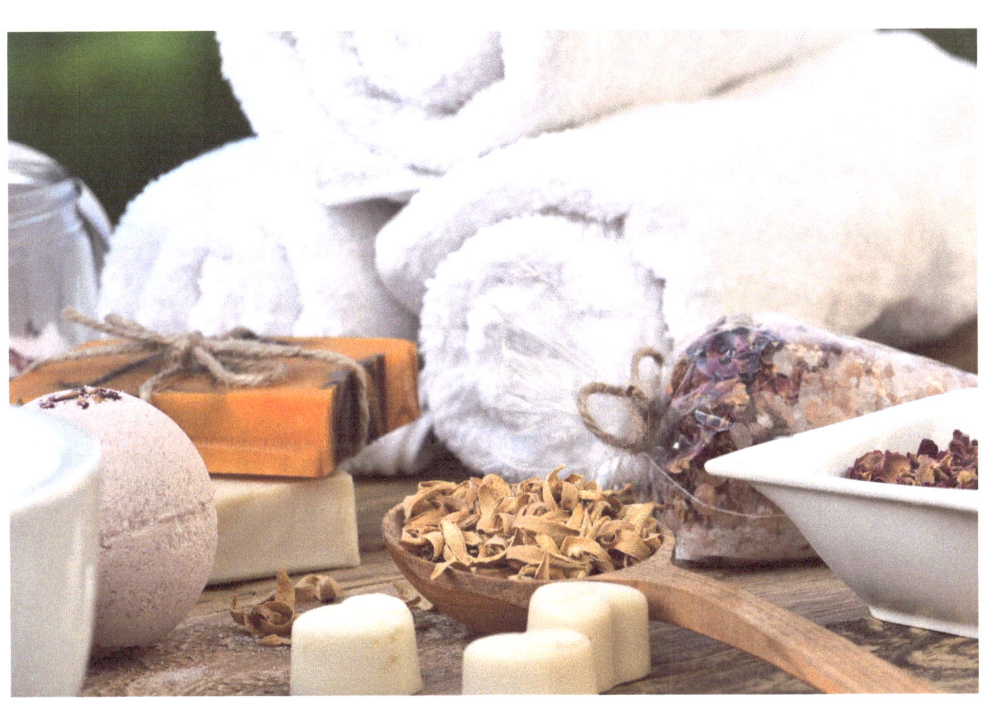

Getting Started

Taking good care of your skin is essential on many levels. It will increase your confidence and ensure your skin is healthy for many years. By using the tips in this book you can fight the aging process on your skin while also reducing dryness, irritation, and other effects of improper skincare.

When you are buying products for your skin, whether your face or body, it's important to know exactly what ingredients are in them. It's possible that many of your skin's imperfections or blemishes are due to the products, and not your skin itself.

Perhaps some of the harsh ingredients being used are causing conditions like rosacea to flare up, or you may be allergic or overly sensitive to some of the ingredients. This can cause redness, itching, hives, burning, and many other negative effects.

The information in this eBook will guide you through the process of switching to a more natural skincare approach. This includes:

Understanding the benefits of a natural skincare routine.

Learning what helps with natural and anti-aging.

Taking care of your body skin and cracked heels.

Learning about dietary changes that can help improve your skin.

Making your own skincare products at home with essential oils and other natural ingredients.

Avoiding toxic chemicals found in many over-the-counter skincare products.

… and more!

Keep reading to learn all about natural skincare and how it can transform your skin to make you look and feel younger and more vibrant.

While there are many do-it-yourself (DIY) skin care products that you can make, natural skincare isn't just about using ingredients you find at home. In many cases, you just want to be careful what ingredients are in the products you put on your face.

It can be tempting to buy the latest lotion or serum you see an advertisement for, but not knowing what is in those products can have disastrous consequences.

For some people, certain chemicals might dry out their skin or increase the risk of blemishes and acne. For others, they may get bad allergic reactions that require a trip to the emergency room.

Perhaps you are using products that are just a little too harsh for your ultra-sensitive skin, or you have a condition like rosacea or eczema where natural is always better.

What Going Natural Means

So, what exactly does "going natural" with your skincare products and treatments mean to you? After reading this book you will have a more defined idea about what going natural means to you and how you personally would like to approach natural skincare.

Going natural can mean something different to everyone. For some it may mean simply being conscientious about the products you put on your skin and making sure they don't contain harsh chemicals. For others it may mean only buying totally natural creams or makeups. Some may even choose to make all their own skincare products themselves. Overall, going natural just means choosing more organic, plant-based ingredients as much as you can. There is no right or wrong method. In this book you will learn that you can still use drugstore or over-the-counter products, but always look at the ingredients list and know what you are putting on your skin. This book will also help you with understanding the labels.

The following chapters are going to go over different ways to switch to a more natural skincare regimen. You'll learn about natural ingredients that fight the aging process and products that fight acne. You'll even see how easy it can be to make your own skincare products!

Chapter 2 – Anti-Aging Tips and Tricks

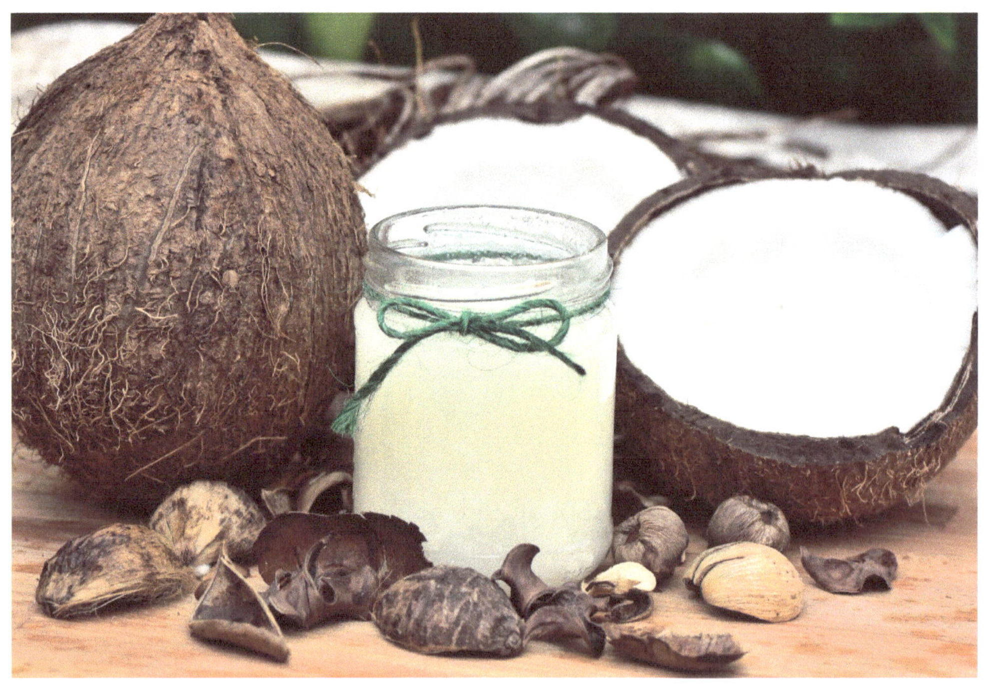

Everyone wants to look younger, and often to go to great lengths to achieve this, but are those expensive treatments and serums really worth it?

Some of them do work very well, but you might also want to look for products that are more natural and less toxic for your skin. The last thing you want to do is do more harm than good in the long run.

While it is good to embrace the natural aging process, the following lifestyle changes and natural remedies can help you age gracefully and in the healthiest way possible.

Drink Plenty of Water

Yes – we are going to start with drinking more water. It may seem like whenever you read health tips, it starts with drinking more water, but that is only because it is essential inside and out.

Not drinking enough water every day can drastically impact your skin, and not in a good way. The amount of water you need to drink often varies based on the article source. Most tell you to try to drink about 8 glasses of water a day.

The best rule of thumb is to drink water when you feel thirsty, and choose it over other drinks like juice and soda.

Don't Smoke

If you already don't smoke, great! You just made this step a lot easier for yourself. However, if you do smoke, it's time to quit or at least cut back. Smoking less can help reduce your chances of developing heart disease, lung cancer, and rapidly aging skin. This is because smoking increases the appearance of wrinkles due to repetitive facial movement.

When you smoke on a regular basis, it often speeds up the aging process, so the best thing you can do for your skin is start cutting back now. Talk to your doctor if you need help quitting, as there are many options available.

Get Regular Exercise

Another good lifestyle habit that can do wonders for your skin and overall anti-aging is to move your body and get the blood flowing.

Regularly exercising and keeping a record of your weight can prevent you from developing chronic health conditions and aging skin. If you exercise every day you can help reduce your symptoms of skin aging, according to Research from McMaster University in Canada. Set aside half an hour to an hour every day to take a walk or head to the gym for a workout. An aerobics workout in your living room from a video is another alternative. Do whatever exercise works for you, but get moving!

Even on days when you're too busy to work out, you can always take the dog for a longer walk in the evening or do some stretches in your bedroom when you wake up in the morning. There are a lot of fun and easy ways to sneak in more exercise during the day, and your body and skin will thank you!

Reduce Your Sugar Intake

According to a 2010 study, researchers found a direct link between dietary sugars and heart disease, obesity, and diabetes. It doesn't mean you are guaranteed to develop these conditions, but it's important to enjoy sugar in limited quantities. Not only does it affect your overall health, but sugar affects your skin. Many skin problems including acne, eczema and rosacea and eczema are exacerbated by eating sugar. Sugar consumption also increases inflammation which breaks down the collagen and elastin in your skin, causing aging affects.

The good news is you don't have to worry so much about natural sugars, like what you find in fresh fruits and vegetables! Instead, simply focus on reducing artificial or added sugar, such as in candy, baked goods, and processed foods. Start reading labels so you can become familiar with how much sugar is in each thing you eat or drink.
If you aren't sure about the exact amount to have each day, talk to your doctor or a nutritionist for recommendations.
Lower Your Stress

Stressful settings can take a serious toll on your mental and physical health. However, keep in mind that stress affects everyone differently. In fact, recent research studies have found that stress can impact people at the cellular level.

Certain types of psychological stress can even wear down a person's body and skin, making it age faster than it would otherwise. However, you can prevent this from happening to you by de-stressing your life with exercise. Just taking a walk can do wonders for you mentally and is great exercise. Begin with a short walk each day if you're just starting your walking routine and gradually increase your time. Make sure to do some leg stretches before you head out on your walk. After a few months you will notice your leg muscles will be stronger and your skin will be firmer!

Here are some easy stress relief ideas:

Spending time with friends and loved ones.
Writing your thoughts in a journal. (Click here for our favorite beach journal and summer journal)
Using essential oils in a diffuser to unwind.
Taking a relaxing bath.
Spending time with pets, which tends to lower your stress levels.
Taking charge of your health is empowering and healthy habits reduce stress. (Click here for a great healthy habits organizer .)

Consume More Protein

It's important that you are eating the proper amount of protein each day. This will help prevent food cravings, help you lose weight, and improve your skin health. According to Keri Gans, RD, protein can help you both build and maintain muscle mass, which people usually lose when they age. By making this small diet change, you can improve the health of your hair, nails, and skin.

Like all dietary changes, it is recommended that you discuss these changes with a doctor before doing anything drastic.

Eat Less Salt

There's no doubt that foods high in sodium make you retain more water, but leave you feeling bloated. At the same time, salty foods can make your face look puffier than normal, especially under your eyes. To prevent this from happening, cut back on salty foods, and instead use lemon, herbs and even fresh peppers and tomatoes to season your food.

To season food, choose spices and herbs instead of excessive salt. Avoid processed or frozen foods as they often are loaded with sodium. Don't use canned foods (especially soups) unless they are low-sodium versions.
If you eat Chinese take-out, ask them to not add MSG (monosodium glutamate.)

Wear Sunscreen

Putting on sunscreen every day is one of the best anti-aging tricks there is. One study from 2013 found that people who wore sunblock at least three or four days a week exhibited fewer signs of aging four and a half years later than those who didn't wear sunscreen.

Continued exposure to the sun can lead to wrinkles and discoloration in the form of dark spots on your face and hands. Even daily UV rays you come into contact with can damage your skin and cause you to age faster. Sunscreen isn't just for the beach; it should be a part of your everyday routine. Even driving in your car on a sunny day can expose your skin to the sun's rays when the sunlight beams through the window.

Cut Down on the Alcohol

Alcohol is naturally dehydrating, so think twice before grabbing another drink at the bar. When your skin is dehydrated, it will look dry, dull, sallow, and crepey. You should be especially careful when drinking white wine. Of all wines, white is most acidic, which means it can damage your teeth's enamel and make them more susceptible to stains. It is also high in sugar content, which can lead to inflammation, cell damage and skin aging.

You don't need to quit completely, unless you want to for other health reasons, but cutting back to just social or special occasion drinking is ideal.

Wash Your Face Before Bed & in the Morning

Washing your face before you go to sleep is crucial for the health of your skin. You must wash off all of the makeup, dirt, and oils that have gathered on your face throughout the day. In fact, failing to wash your face at the end of the night actually inhibits your skin's ability to regenerate overnight. Plus, you don't want to wake up with clogged pores, pimples and blackheads.

Washing your face when you get up in the morning is also extremely important. Exfoliate with a soapy washcloth to remove oil, dirt and dead skin cells.

Make sure you choose your facial products wisely, reading labels for natural ingredients instead of toxic and harsh chemicals. Glycerin based soaps made from palm oil or coconut oil are great for oily or combination skin as they have a slight drying effect. This can reduce pimple break outs and blemishes and give your face a healthy glow. Also look for glycerin in toners or astringents.

Change Your Pillowcase

Changing your pillowcase frequently is sometimes overlooked as part of keeping your skin free from acne and pimples. Oils from our face and hair, combined with sweat and dust can build up quickly on our pillowcases. Changing your pillowcase often can prevent breakouts from happening.

Get a Good Night's Sleep

Sleep is an essential and often overlooked part of your regular skincare routine. It is so incredibly important because it helps the body and the skin to regenerate. Getting the recommended eight hours of sleep every night will help your skin cells rebuild. Plus, it will also prevent dark under-eye circles.

With a few lifestyle changes and a better diet, you can continue to look young for a long time to come. By taking advantage of the tips above, you can prevent the signs of aging naturally. From your skin to your teeth, you will be looking younger in no time at all.

Natural Anti-Aging Moisturizers

Coconut oil (which is solid at room temperature) is a wonderfully natural anti-aging moisturizer for your face. It smooths out wrinkles and fine facial lines and strengthens the connective tissues, actually tightening your skin! Coconut oil helps the cells produce collagen and boosts cell regeneration. Finally, it has antioxidants that prevent premature skin aging. It works wonders without the expense of factory made creams.

Also on the list of anti-aging moisturizers are almond oil, shea butter, olive oil, rose hip oil, and carrot seed oil. Vitamins A, C and E also help repair damage from the sun, firm the skin and smooth fine lines. These vitamins can also help lessen the appearance of stretch marks.

With a few lifestyle changes and a better diet, you can continue to look young for a long time to come. By taking advantage of the tips above, you can prevent the signs of aging naturally. From your skin to your teeth, you will be looking younger in no time at all.

Chapter 3 – What You Eat Affects Your Skin

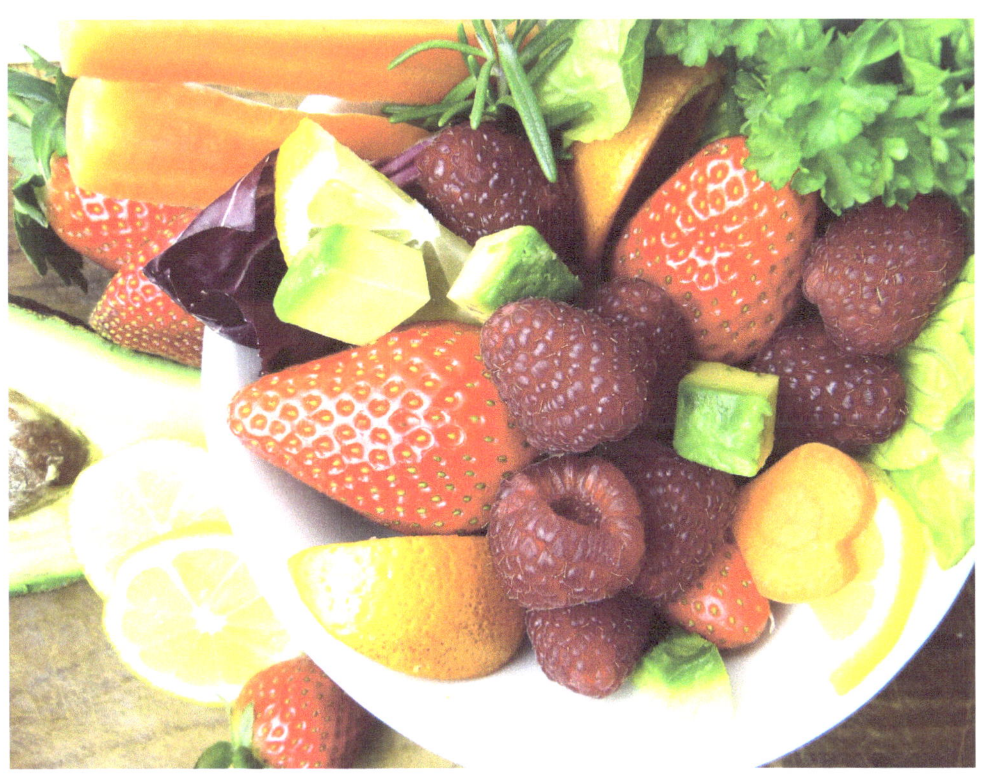

Aging is a fact of life. Wrinkles and spots are natural and will show up with time, but it is possible to slow them and reduce the appearance of wrinkles and fine lines on the face. Similarly, it is also possible to clear up acne by keeping focused on what goes into our bodies. There are many factors that go affect skin health such as lifestyle habits and heredity, but nutrition also plays a large role.

If you want to keep your skin young and healthy looking for as long as possible, you need to focus on what you eat. Below is a look at some of the factors in the relationship between your diet and skin health.

Good Vs Bad Fats

Fat is an important part of your diet and is crucial for good skin health. Your body uses fat as a waterproof seal and healthy fats help to improve the health of your skin.

For optimal skin health, you should consume adequate amounts of Omega-3 fatty acids and omega-6 fatty acids. Good sources of Omega 3 can be found in fatty fish, walnuts, flaxseeds, chia seeds, soybeans, and tofu. Some eggs are also omega-3 enriched. Omega 6 is also found in nuts and seeds, meat, fish, olives and whole grains.

Keep in mind that a meat-heavy diet increases the amount of animal fat that you consume. Excessive consumption of animal fat can lead to more free radicals being produced in your body, which can have negative effects on your skin at the cellular level. Your skin does need some fat, but you should stick to the healthy types such as those from fatty fish, olives and nuts. In addition to preventing dry skin, good fats help your body to absorb antioxidants and vitamins. Consuming healthy fats can also strengthen your cell membranes.

Vitamins

Vitamin C is essential for healthy skin. Vitamins C works together with vitamin E to prevent damage to skin cells due to sun exposure. In addition, your skin's structure depends on a protein called collagen. Vitamin C helps your body to produce the collagen you need to keep your skin cells strong and healthy. Collagen is what gives your skin its elasticity and plays a role in keeping your skin hydrated. As you get older your body does not produce as much collagen, which leads to dry skin and wrinkles. So, keeping up with your vitamin C intake is essential.

Of course, another important benefit of vitamin C is that it helps to support your immune system. A healthy immune system may help keep you healthy, especially in the winter. A robust immune system can also speed up the healing process for blemishes.

To make sure you're getting enough vitamin C, be sure your diet includes fruits and vegetables high in vitamin C. Besides citrus fruits, high amounts of vitamin C are found in cantaloupe, pineapple, strawberries, raspberries, blueberries and watermelon. Vegetables high in vitamin C include red peppers, Brussels sprouts and broccoli.

Processed Foods

Studies of certain primitive cultures with diets that consist mostly of fish, fruit and tubers (underground plants such as potatoes, carrots, beets, radishes, turnips, etc.) with almost no processed foods, have shown no incidences of acne. Researchers believe that this is because processed foods like refined carbohydrates cause the release of hormones that produce more skin oils and slough off skin cells. Those skin cells clog pores and result in acne.

While genetics may play a role in healthy skin, research has also shown that members of these populations who move to areas where western-style diets are consumed do develop acne. Therefore, we know diet is a main factor in skin health.

Dairy

Research has shown that the consuming dairy increases the extent of an acne outbreak as well as its severity. Dairy is full of hormones like testosterone and insulin- the same hormones that processed foods are believed to trigger. Consuming dairy can increase insulin by as much as 300 percent.

Hydration

Like the other cells in your body, skin cells consist mostly of water. Insufficient hydration will result in your skin cells not performing properly.

Among water's benefits is the fact that it increases the blood flow of capillaries in the skin thus increasing the skin's elasticity. While there is no evidence to support the notion that extra water consumption increases skin health, the research does show that insufficient hydration can detract from it.

What is going on the outside of your body directly reflects what is happening on the inside. Eating a diet with natural foods and staying hydrated will ensure healthy skin, but a diet full of processed foods will deprive your skin of the nutrients and hormonal stability needed for optimal health.

Omega-3

Fish oil is high in Omega-3 and is proven to clear up skin that has broken out in pimples. Ask your doctor about taking fish oil capsules to clear up your skin, whether its your face, shoulders, arms or back that has a breakout. It may take 6 weeks to see the effects but it will be well worth it to see those problem spots disappear.

Vitamin A

Vitamin A is great for the skin both topically and as a supplement. (Make sure to check with your doctor before taking any supplements, and to get correct dosage amounts.) Vitamin A can keep your skin clear and blemish-free with its antioxidant power and anti-inflammatory properties. Like Omega-3, results may take a few weeks, but you will see a huge difference if your skin is prone to breakouts.

Chapter 4 - DIY Skincare Products with Essential Oils

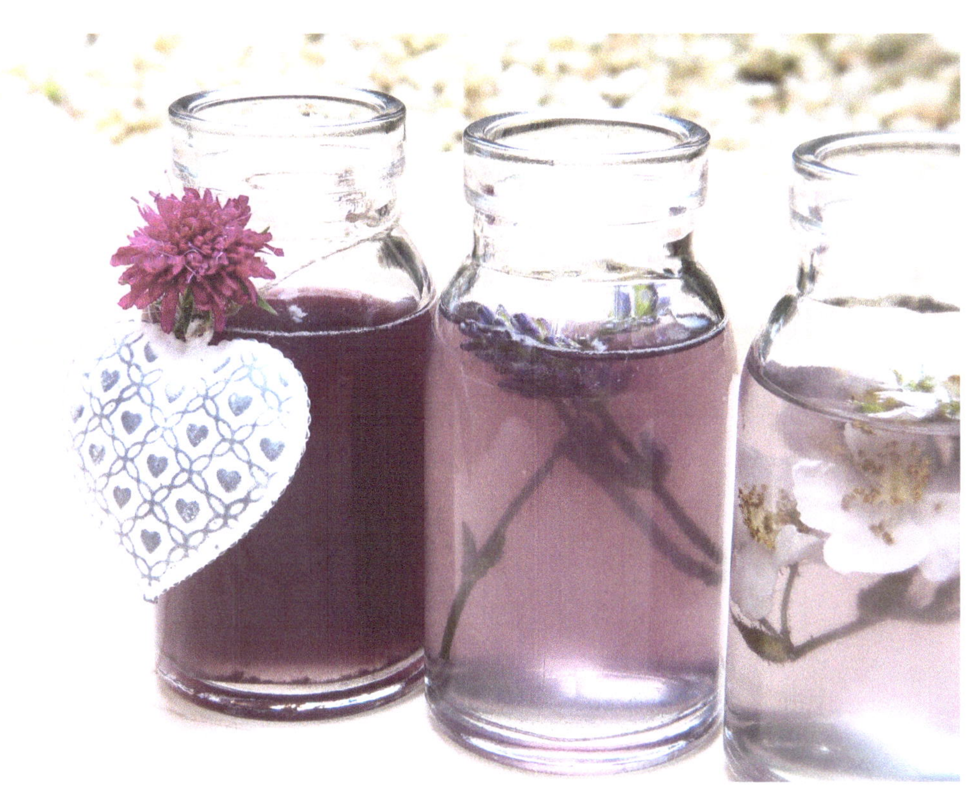

Why not start going natural by making your own skincare products? DIY ("Do it Yourself") products are great since many base ingredients are already in your kitchen and then you can add essential oils for multiple benefits. Making your own skincare products allows you to use the most pure and natural ingredients possible while customizing them for your exact skin type. Not to mention they are fun to make, either by yourself, with friends or with kids! The also make extra special gifts!

You can make everything from scratch: soap, toners, lotions, scrubs and more. Also, so as to not forget the gentlemen, you can also make beard oils to tame unruly beard hair while also hydrating the skin underneath so ingrown hairs become less common. The possibilities are endless and there is something for everyone.

To get started, first determine your skin type. Then read about the essential oils below to decide which ones are best for you. If you plan to make gifts for others, it is also a good idea to ask them about their skin type beforehand and use this book as a guide as to which ingredients to use.

Essential Oils for Certain Skin Types

We all have different skin types, so it's useful to know which oils will be best for the skin you have. Some are great for balancing skin while others protect and nourish aging skin. A few skin types are extremely common: oily, dry, combination, blemish prone, and aging. Many people also have more than one skin problem. For example, a person could have both dry and aging skin or oily and dry (combination skin.)

<u>Essential Oils for Oily Skin:</u>

Orange
Lemon
Lime
Bergamot
Geranium
Cypress

Essential Oils for Dry Skin:

<u>Chamomile</u>
<u>Cedarwood</u>
<u>Geranium</u>
<u>Myrrh</u>
<u>Palmarosa</u>

Essential Oils for Acne-Prone Skin:

Lavender
Geranium
Vetiver
Patchouli

Essential Oils for Aging Skin:

Tangerine
Ylang Ylang
Frankincense
Lavender
Rose, Rosemary, Rose Hip, Rose Geranium
Palmarosa
Sandalwood
Carrot seed
Pomegranite seed
Lemon
Clary Sage

Making Skincare Products with Essential Oils

Now that you know which essential oils will work for your skin, you can decide which products would benefit you. You can make many skincare products at home without spending a fortune. Here are a few:

Lotion

There are a few simple ingredients that you will need to make your own lotion with essential oils. Shea butter is common as a base, and you can add essential oils that work with your specific skin type. For instance, if you have aging skin, try adding tangerine or rose oil to nourish skin that is beginning to sag and have wrinkles. If your skin is prone to being both dry and oily, you can try adding lavender.

Toners

Toners are great for removing excess soap and makeup and balancing skin. They also leave facial skin feeling velvety soft. Witch hazel is an ingredient often added to toners for oily or blemish-prone skin, as it has a balancing effect on the oil. For dry or aging skin, toners are usually made are made solely from essential oils best suited for those skin types.

Serums

Serums help brighten and moisturize the skin white decreasing dark circles under the eyes. For serums, a carrier oil, such as jojoba oil, is used as the base and essential oils are added according to your skin type. For instance, a person who needs a solution for wrinkles but also has dry skin might add small amounts of rose oil and chamomile to jojoba oil to make their serum.

Beard Oils

Men often have many of the same skin problems that women have, and they benefit from many of the products like lotions and toners. Many men, however, also have beards to care for.

Beard oil softens beard hair while also nourishing the skin underneath. A carrier oil, such as coconut oil, is often used as a base, and a masculine smelling essential oil that is suited to the skin type of the user is added in.

Eucalyptus is an essential oil that is also an antiseptic and can treat acne. It also has a clean, fresh scent that isn't too feminine. Sandalwood is another scent that has a woodsy, masculine scent. It's great in a beard oil because of its moisturizing effect. Another essential oil that works great for men is lemon oil. This particular oil is great for oily skin as it cuts oil production.

Lip Balms

Lip balms are another skincare product that almost anyone can benefit from. Common ingredients are beeswax, shea butter, coconut oil, lavender oil, and peppermint oil. You can also add in a pigmentation such as beet juice if you would like to have a rosy tint that can substitute for lipstick. Natural recipes are often preferred by people because it's very common to accidentally ingest products that we put on our mouths.

Essential oils not only help improve the quality of your skin without harsh chemicals, but they also, oftentimes, smell great. While you shouldn't choose your essential oils based solely on the fragrance, there are many options available for whatever skin issues that you are trying to regulate, so you are sure to find something that not only works great, but is also pleasing to you.

Soap

All true soap contains lye. However, if you want to make natural soap at home without handling the lye, there are many natural "melt and pour" soap bases available, such as honey or goats' milk varieties available online or in craft stores. You simply cut the soap and melt it along with any additives you want- honey, bath salts, herbs, essential oils, etc. Pour into a mold and *voila!* You have your own homemade natural soap! Homemade soap always makes a great gift!

Scrubs

Facial scrubs are exfoliants to slough away dead skin cells and freshen your face naturally. The problem with many facial scrubs in the drugstores is that many contain tiny plastic beads to exfoliate your skin, which are then washed down the drain and pollute the environment. For all-natural exfoliants, just raid your kitchen cabinets! You can make "delicious" (but not edible) scrubs with one or more of the following ingredients: oatmeal, brown sugar and honey, baking soda, and even coffee grounds! Simply blend a small amount into a teaspoon of essential oil for a facial scrub that will rival any spa treatment but from the comfort of your home! Because you're worth it!

Chapter 5 - Banish Cracked Heels for Good

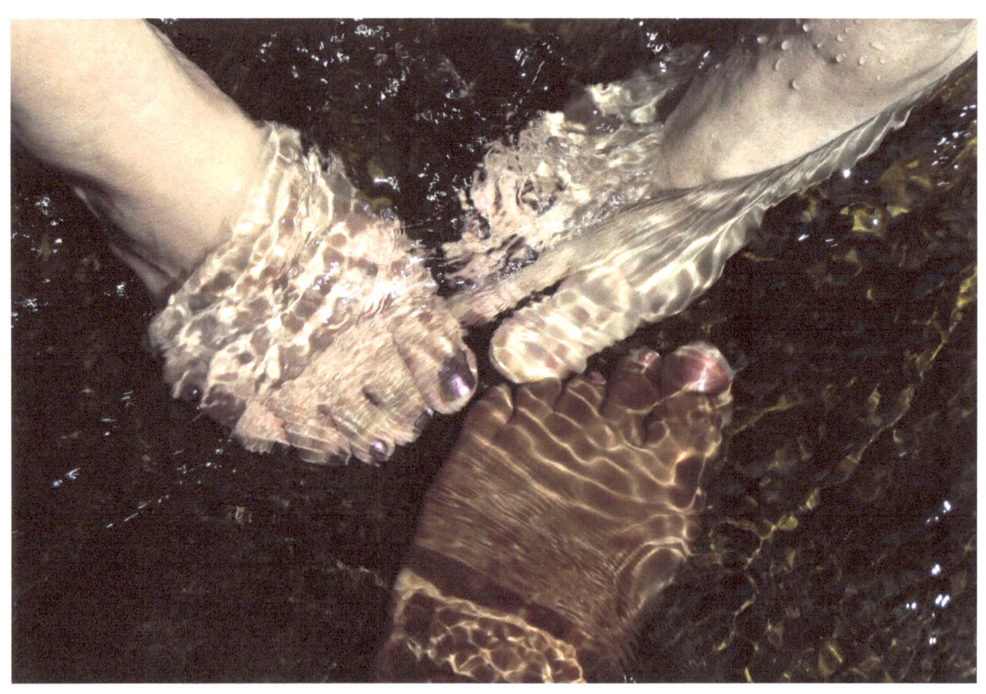

You know that feeling, when the heels of your feet are so dry it's discomforting. Some people don't want anyone to even see their feet because it looks so dry and cracked. If this is you, you're not alone! It is estimated that about 20 percent of adults in the U.S. suffer from cracked heels.

It's great to get a pedicure or foot treatment at your local spa, but why not try healing your cracked heels at home? Here are some natural remedies that can work wonders:

Penetrating Oils

Cracked heels do not happen overnight. It is the result of ignoring the skin on your heels over time.

Layers of severely dry skin crack under pressure. You need to use something that can penetrate the layers like coconut oil or other organic oils. Wash your feet, pat them dry, use a pumice stone to exfoliate, and apply the oil. Put on clean socks to leave the oil on overnight and repeat these steps for a few days.

Gentle Exfoliation

Those with layers of dead skin may want to consider exfoliating. Sure, using a pumice stone works, but it may not be enough when the problem is extensive. You may need a specialized exfoliating solution to help deal with your specific foot problem. You can mix a specific natural blend meant to exfoliate but also medicate the region.

What you want to do is start with a handful of ground rice. Begin to add a few teaspoons of raw honey and unpasteurized apple cider vinegar to the rice until you get a paste-like consistency.

Add a few teaspoons of your choice of oil. Soak your feet in lukewarm water for about 10 minutes, and then scrub with the solution. Do this for about a week or until you're satisfied with how your heels feel.
 Leafy Aid

Cracked feet comes in many forms depending on the severity of the condition. Some that just have mild cracks and discomfort while others have severe symptoms like infections or itchiness. It is important to apply a more poignant solution when your cracked feet are this severe, like this leafy solution.

For the most severe cases of cracked feet, use neem leaves (also known as margosa or Indian lilac.) Crush the leaves with a teaspoon of turmeric powder and add a little water to make a paste. Blend well, and apply it to the affected areas. Keep the paste on for 30 minutes, and then rinse your feet and pat dry. The neem will naturally soothe your feet and also effectively kills fungus.

Lemony Softness

Lemons are known for their natural acidic properties, which is helpful for your cracked heels. The acidic active ingredients in lemon should help soften the skin given enough time. Don't apply the lemon directly but rather dilute it so that it's not too aggressive.

Mix lemon juice from one lemon into enough water to soak your feet. Again, you want to use lukewarm water, not hot water, which could exasperate dryness. Let your feet soak in the warm water for 10 to 15 minutes before scrubbing them with a pumice stone. End by rinsing and pat drying your feet.

Rosy Wash

Another effective solution comes from the combination of glycerin and rose water. There are a few reasons why this solution is helpful. Glycerin, for one, helps to soften the skin like lemon but is not as aggressive. Rose water contains a lot of skin-strengthening ingredients like vitamin A, B3, C, E, and antioxidants just to name a few.

You should simply mix both of these solutions in equal parts and apply to your clean feet. Make sure you let the blend stay on your feet overnight, so wear clean socks or wraps around your feet. Do this a number of times until the condition gets better.

Banana Goodness

One of the most interesting and inexpensive solutions is the banana-based one. Bananas have strong moisturizing properties, and you are going to be using these properties to help you deal with your cracked heels. All you have to do is mash a banana and apply a healthy layer over the affected areas.

Now, your feet need to be clean and dry before you apply the paste. Let the banana mush sit over the affected areas for 10 to 15 minutes before washing it off. Make sure that you do this every day for a week or until your skin feels better.

Hopefully, some of these solutions help you find relief. Be sure to pass them on because they are effective and can help others in your situation. You could also talk to your podiatrist to see if he or she has additional suggestions.

Chapter 6 - Natural Skincare Tips for Your Body

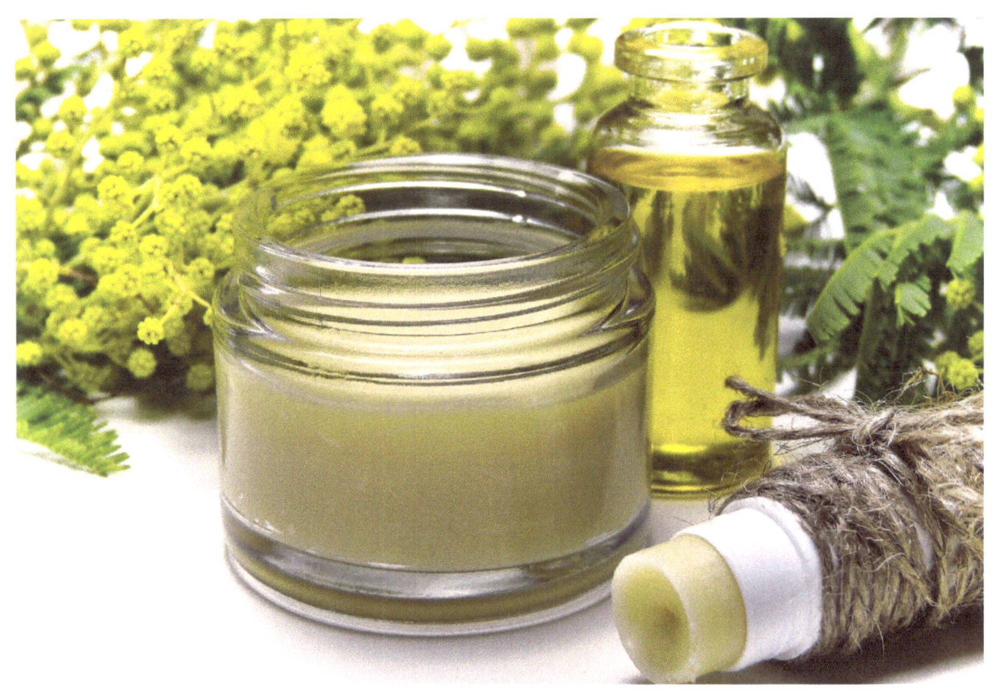

Caring for your skin is one of the most important things you can do for yourself. You only get the skin you're born with, and caring for it is the best way to feel more confident, more beautiful, and to prevent telltale signs of obvious aging from prematurely occurring. Your skin is exposed to so many elements on a daily basis it would shock you to break them down individually, and caring for it daily helps minimize the effects of everyday life.

Before you assume the only way to care for your skin is through the use of expensive products, here are a few of the simplest, most natural ways to care for your skin all over your body. You can do it at home, and you can live a healthier, more beautiful life.

Natural Skincare for Your Entire Body

Before delving into the specifics of caring for each individual body part, it's imperative you learn what you can do naturally at home to improve your skin as a whole. The most important thing you can do is drink more water. Your body is comprised of mostly water, and you must replenish it daily. The more water you drink, the healthier your skin looks.

Drinking enough water prevents dehydration, and it can even improve the overall look of your skin. It improves your collagen, which is what keeps your skin looking healthy and happy. It also helps you clear up breakouts and other imperfections on your face. Water is the healthiest thing you can consume, and it shows in your skin's glow.

Another great way to improve the look of your skin overall is to eat a healthy, balanced diet. There's no need to deprive yourself of the many things you love, but there is a good reason to eat healthy foods. It helps keep your weight in check, it helps your skin look better, and it makes you look and feel healthier. Finally, you must get enough sleep.

Adults need 7 to 8 hours of sleep per night to function at your highest capacity, which means you need to adjust your bed time and/or wakeup time to allow your body the sleep it needs.

Natural Skincare for Your Face

Did you know you can wash your face with Apple Cider Vinegar a few times a week to help your skin look clearer and more beautiful? To use it as a natural astringent, all you need to do is dip a cotton ball into apple cider vinegar, squeeze off the excess, and wipe the cotton ball all over your face. Be sure to not get it in your eyes! It's all natural, safe, will clear breakouts and improve the overall look of your skin.

Exfoliate Your Elbows, Knees and Ankles!

If you want to avoid dry, crusty spots on your main joints, you must exfoliate regularly. A routine of exfoliating every other day is best. One way to do this is with a mixture of sea salt, sugar and a touch of olive oil. It will remove dead skin from your elbows, knees and ankles while moisturizing them along the way.

Take Care of Your Legs and Feet

Your legs and feet take the brunt the abuse. They're the body parts getting the most sun, and they're the body parts that end up more damaged than any other part. Think of all the beautiful shoes you wear that leave blisters and marks on your feet. That's damage to your skin even if it's not something you think of often.

Your legs will thank you for using a very simple homemade skincare routine on them every day. All you need is a little coconut oil. Rub it on your legs every time you get out of the shower. Consider this as your new moisturizer! It's one of the best ways to combat dry skin and damaged skin on your legs.

As for your feet, the most important thing you can do is prevent cracking and dryness. We seem to accept cracked feet as natural, but it's not natural. Your skin shouldn't get to this point, but it does when you're not spending enough time caring for the skin on your feet. A pumice stone is a great way to combat this problem.

For extra dry feet, rub in a little coconut oil and wear socks to bed a few times a month. This helps set in moisture naturally, and makes that dry, uncomfortable skin look and feel smoother and healthier.

Chapter 7 - Chemicals to Avoid

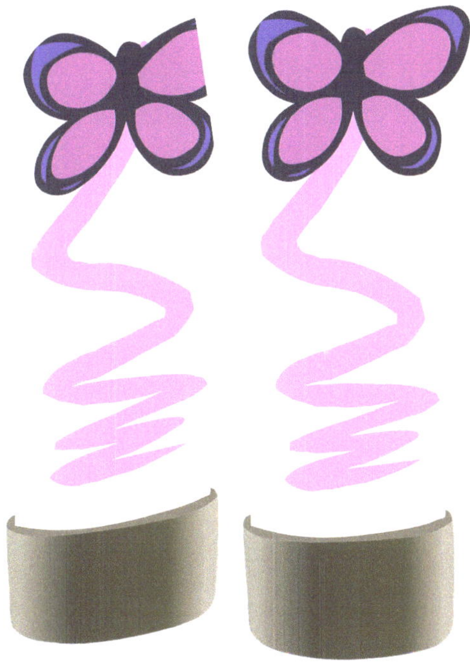

Many drugstore skincare products contain harsh chemicals that consumers with sensitive skin need to avoid. As published in the article, "Dangerous Ingredients in Skin Care Products," on Natural Health Source's website, more than 10,000 dangerous ingredients are used to manufacture beauty products. Considering these staggering statistics, consumers should be careful when selecting products to use on their skin. In this industry that is largely unregulated for practical purposes, consumers are forced to fend for themselves.

The best way shoppers can protect themselves is to read the list of ingredients to make an informed decision. Unfortunately, deceptive labeling practices make it almost impossible to simply scan the label since positive words like "natural" are indiscriminately used to bolster a product's image, but may not be correct.

Even when a product is labeled organic, there is still a risk since the requirement for using the word organic is that the item must have at least 70 percent organic ingredients. What that means is that, effectively, 30 percent of the product is "not organic."

Listed below are some of the worst offenders.

1. Parabens

Parabens are used because they add to the shelf life of products, acting as a preservative by preventing the growth of bacteria and fungi. It is noteworthy that research has found parabens present in breast cancer tissue. Skin allergies are also common. When trying to identify parabens, the prefixes propyl, methyl and butyl are tip offs. To be on the safe side, it is always a good idea to look for and buy paraben-free products.

2. Propylene Glycol

This ingredient is tied to liver and kidney health problems. Additionally, it is considered an allergen. It is no surprise that this chemical compound is dangerous when you consider its other use as a plane de-icing agent.

3. PEG Compounds

These compounds are often present in skin creams. The dioxane in this compound is believed to cause cancer. Consumers should steer clear of ingredients with "eth" in the name to avoid exposure.

4. BHT and BHI

These two chemicals have been found to be harmful to wildlife and humans. Often present in moisturizers, they are tied to cancer and should always be avoided.

5. Fragrances

Consumers should shop for fragrance-free products to avoid some of the nasty symptoms commonly connected to these (parfum) additives. Headaches and rashes are two frequent unpleasant side effects. Vomiting and dizziness have also been reported and associated with those manufactured smells the chemists work so hard to add to beauty products.

6. Phthalates

This chemical is often one of the ingredients you'll often find in lotion. If you see phthalates as an ingredient, beware. They are tied to serious health issues that include liver and kidney damage. Phthalates are also linked to cancer and lung damage.

7. DEA and TEA

These two compounds are particularly dangerous and should be avoided whenever possible. Found in body wash and soaps, a few of the more minor problems consumers can expect include dry skin and hair. Eye irritations have also been reported. The problems only get more serious from there. Commonly used in moisturizers, these ingredients are believed to cause organ damage, specifically in the liver and kidneys.

8. Formaldehyde-Related Preservatives

Consumers need to be on the alert for these preservatives. As recognized carcinogens, DMDM and methenamine must be added to the list of dangerous additives to avoid. Hydantoin and quarternium-15 are also believed to increase cancer levels and are commonly found in popular cosmetic brands.

9. Mineral Oil

This may be one of the least likely to make a list of toxins, but it definitely deserves to be avoided. This petroleum by-product is found in many moisturizers and clogs the skin. Since the skin is charged with the important function of releasing toxins, clogged skin inhibits its ability to do so.

10. Petrolatum

As the name suggests, this is a petroleum product. It is found in many moisturizers. The problem with this chemical is that it is linked to a higher risk of cancer, so avoid it.

While this list is by no means exhaustive, it represents the most frequently used chemicals that health-conscious consumers need to eliminate from their skincare products.

Since beauty and health related products are not as regulated as is necessary to truly protect the public, the burden of keeping their families safe rests largely on the consumer's shoulders when selecting skincare products.

The more ingredients listed on a product, the more likely it is to contain one of these toxic chemicals. Considering the sheer number of chemicals the average person is exposed to on a daily basis, anything a consumer can do to eliminate toxins that enter the body makes sense.

Armed with knowledge, consumers are positioned to proactively purchase skincare products that will enhance their life and health with no associated risks.

Chapter 8 - Natural Skincare Ingredients

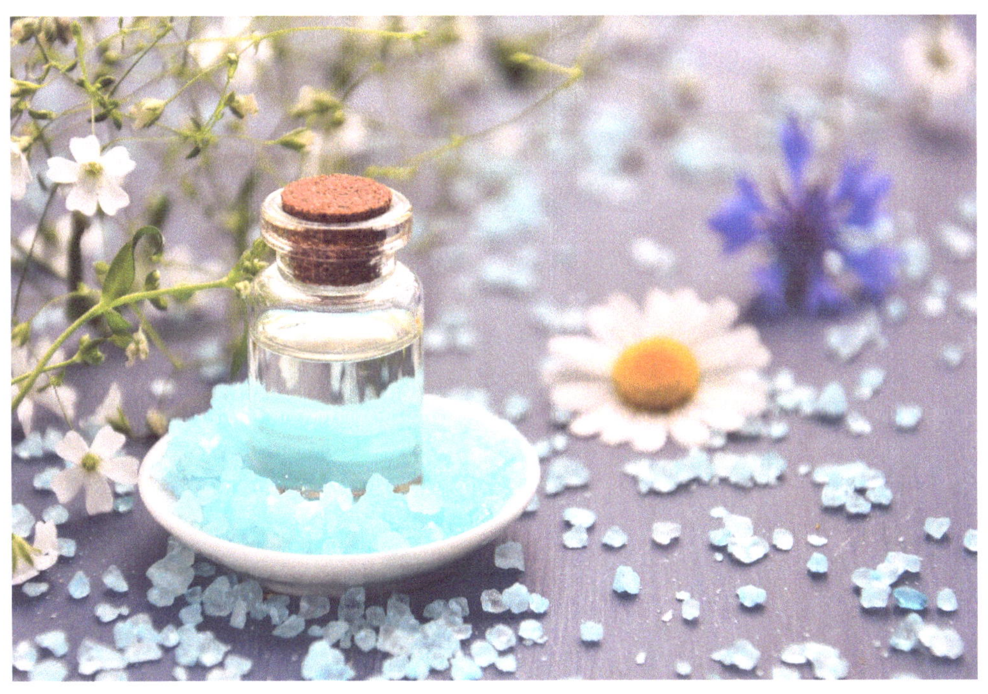

A big part of looking young is having good skin. Your skin represents your age, and you should take care of it like you would anything else. Sadly, many commercial skincare products do more harm than good. Makeup and other facial products can clog your pores, resulting in acne or blemishes which can leave scars. With all that being said, there are still many products available that *are* good for your skin. Most of the time, these products will be natural and won't be filled with lots of extra ingredients. In this article, we will discuss some of the most recommended natural skincare products.

Coconut Oil

Coconut is one of the most useful skin care products available and is great for the skin. It contains Vitamins A and E along with anti-microbial properties that can help treat acne, moisturize, remove makeup. It is great as a body moisturizer as well. Just use as you would any body oil after a shower on wet skin, then pat dry. You will smell like you just got back from the beach! Use a dab of coconut oil to smooth fine lines around the eyes or use as an anti-aging overnight cream to combat wrinkles.

Coconut oil can be used on the scalp and hair for numerous benefits. On the scalpt can help treat the worst cases of dandruff. Just a small amount is an effective leave-in hair moisturizer and frizz tamer!

Due to all the wide range of benefits that coconut oil provides, it is at the top of the list as far as skin care products go.

Tea Tree Oil

Tea tree oil is great for skincare because it reduces inflammation and redness. It also provides relief from breakouts. It is helpful for skin problems such as acne, psoriasis and eczema.

Tea Tree Oil even has the power to treat warts and athletes foot. For maximum results, you will need a high-quality product. While lots of lotions and cleansers have a small amount of tea tree oil in them, they may not be as effective as 100% tea tree oil.
Use a small amount directly on the skin for best results. Tea Tree Oil is relatively inexpensive and can be found easily online.

Avocado

Avocado is another powerful option for natural skin care. Avocado is filled with tons of antioxidants like alpha-carotene and beta-carotene. All of these antioxidants are great for effectively fighting off bacteria on the skin. It is also useful for diminishing wrinkles preventing signs of aging. Avocado also has Vitamins E and C which act together to protect and heal the skin.

Along with Coconut Oil, Avocado is good for consuming as well. Eating Avocado can help your skin just as products with Avocado in them can. It has fatty acids which help your skin look younger and healthier. Avocado also has moisturizing properties which are necessary for healing dry or cracked skin.

Raw Honey

You may wonder why honey has made the list as a natural skincare product. Although the thought of putting honey on your skin may sound messy, it can actually be beneficial.

Honey contains antibacterial and probiotic properties that are great for your skin. It also has extreme hydrating powers. Although honey won't be good for removing your makeup, it does make a great cleanser.

Simply wet your face and apply a little dab of honey. Massage it into your face like you would any other cleansers. The water will also ensure that you won't make a sticky mess in the process. After you wash it off, your skin will be smooth, hydrated, and protected from bacteria.

All in all, honey is great for your skin whether you use it topically or if you eat it! Topically might be the best choice though, as the large amounts of sugar found in honey could lead to breakouts.

Sea Salt

Sea Salt is very useful for healthy skin, hair, teeth, and even nails! When it comes to skincare specifically, there are many reasons why sea salt is beneficial. One of the biggest reasons is because sea salt is filled with minerals like magnesium and calcium. Many of the minerals found in sea salt play a key role in skin health.

There are many ways to use sea salt for your skin. You can use it as a mask by mixing it with honey. You can use it as a toner as well. Sea salt helps regulate the production of oil and bacteria on the skin which can fend off breakouts. You can also use sea salt as a facial scrub. Sea salt has a gritty texture which can be great for getting deep into your pores and removing dead skin cells.

Aloe Vera

Aloe Vera is another natural skin care product that you can use to enhance your skin. The first thing that comes to mind when people think of Aloe Vera is treating sunburns.

Aloe Vera has powerful moisturizing and healing abilities when it comes to the skin. Many people find that this is one of the best remedies for treating a sunburn. It turns out that there are many other practical uses for Aloe Vera as well, including treating acne, fighting aging, and reducing the appearance of stretch marks. Aloe Vera contains strong anti-inflammatory ingredients like Auxin and Gibberellins which fight acne. It also contains vitamins and antioxidants which are great for reducing the signs of aging and stretch marks.

Cocoa Butter

Cocoa butter comes from cocoa beans- the same beans used to make chocolate. It is rich in antioxidants, fatty acids and vitamins that moisturize and improve the elasticity of the skin, which can help with stretch marks during pregnancy. Plus, it has that naturally delicious cocoa aroma!

Chapter 9 - Seasonal Skincare Tips

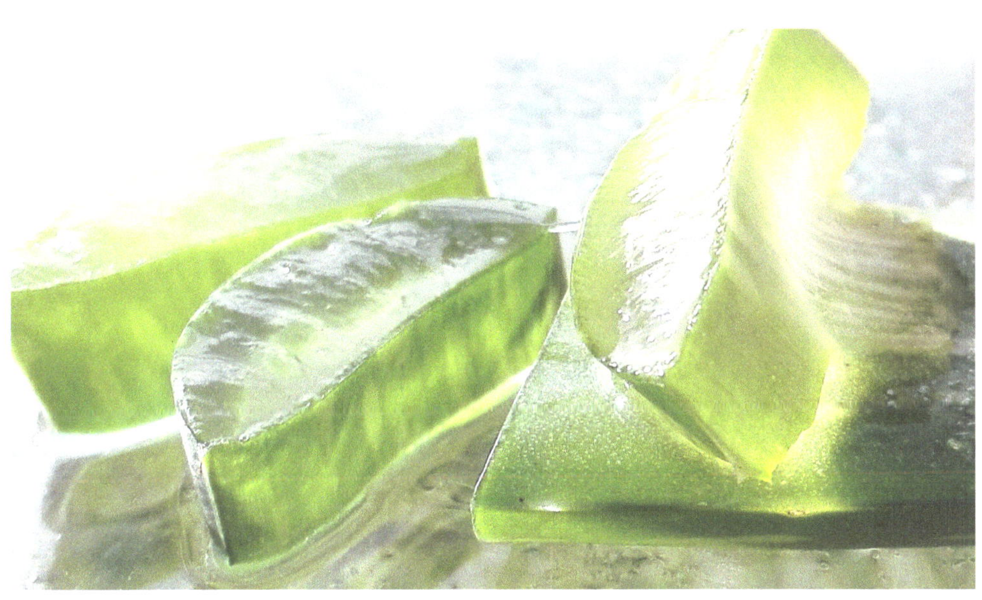

There are so many options when it comes to taking care of your skin. Although there are numerous products, it is very important to make sure that everything you put on your skin is as non-toxic as possible.

The skin is the body's biggest organ and easily absorbs anything put onto it, including any toxins such as parabens, synthetic fragrances, and dyes.

One of the easiest ways to ensure that your skin doesn't become a hotbed of toxins is to use as many natural options as possible. And throughout the seasons, the skin requires different ways of taking care of it for it to operate in peak condition.

Spring

Exfoliate

Springtime calls for renewal and the spring clean-up. That should be true for your skin as well. When transitioning your skin from winter to spring, one of the most important things to do is to exfoliate.

There are many products with which this can be achieved, but the natural way is usually much easier, cheaper, and more forgiving on the skin. Simply mix raw sugar, ground coffee, and roughly ground oatmeal with coconut oil to create a simple paste that will be extremely effective in exfoliating the skin.

Antioxidants

Springtime also brings about more time in the sun, which means your skin will be more exposed to the ultraviolet rays it gives off. First, make sure to use sunscreen when out in the sun. At night, combat the effects of the sun naturally with an essential oil, such as lavender or carrot seed oil, both of which work to reverse the effects of the sun's harmful rays on the skin.

More time in the sun means your skin will also benefit from more antioxidants in your diet. Antioxidants work to reverse the signs of sun damage. For added antioxidants, be sure to add berries and leafy greens to get to your diet!

Sensitive Skin

The sensitive skin around the eyes also needs to be protected more in the spring. Many people make the mistake of thinking they don't need their sunglasses yet in the spring, and the skin under your eyes suffers. Creating a simple eye cream with shea butter and frankincense essential oil will keep that delicate portion of the skin in peak condition.

Summer

Sun Care

Summer is the time to really pay attention to the effects that the sun has on your skin. Carrot seed oil, raspberry seed oil, coconut oil and sesame seed oil work well as natural alternatives to conventional sunscreen. They contain a natural SPF of 35 to 40.

Still, to keep your skin in peak condition, limit time in the sun to about an hour at a time and make sure to reapply the natural SPF about every half hour. Shade and protective clothing are also musts for the health of your skin.

After Sun Care

Should you happen to get sunburned from too much sun, there are a few natural ways to diminish the effects of the sunburn and to keep your skin more comfortable until it heals.

Aloe Vera gel is always the go-to for these situations. Use pure gel without any added chemicals or ingredients. For these times it's good to always have an Aloe Vera plant in your home on the windowsill to lend you a leaf when you need it. You can also use peppermint oil for a cooling effect on the skin.

Moisturize

The extra heat can also be drying to the skin, so make sure that you have a good moisturizer handy. Coconut oil works well to keep your skin hydrated. If you normally have acne-prone or oily skin, opt for adding just a few drops of coconut oil to another moisturizer to thin it out before applying it to your face. This will ensure you are getting the proper amount of moisture to your skin and will keep it from the drying affects of the intense heat.

Fall

Keep Moisturizing

During the fall, the wind is usually playing all kinds of havoc with your hair, but don't forget about your skin. Take care to keep extra moisturized during this time, as the wind has a very drying effect on the skin, especially skin on your face.
Continuing with coconut oil as a moisturizer is a good way to keep your skin healthy. Also, take extra care of the skin on your hands at this time in the season as it usually gets much dryer than usual.

Exfoliate Again

The fall season calls for another good round of exfoliation. This is the best time for it because the weather stays in temperatures that are less extreme on either end so a freshly exposed skin on your face won't have as many temperature fluctuations to deal with.

Again, a natural, homemade scrub is the easiest and least toxic one to use. Make sure to add some moisture back in along with the scrub. The best way is to add a super moisturizing oil, such as grapeseed oil, into your scrub. Don't just limit exfoliating to your face either, your whole body needs it during these months.

Facial Masks

A good step to add to a beauty routine during the fall is use a facial mask. Masks will deliver a lot of nutrients, vitamins, and benefits to your skin and will help prep your skin for the coming winter months. Make sure to choose masks with ingredients that are suited to the skin on your face. If you're looking for a mask to help turn back the signs of aging or to brighten your face, opt for a yogurt and lemon juice mask.

Those who want something moisturizing and luxurious for their face, along with the nutritional benefits, should try masks with avocado, banana, honey or aloe vera gel.

Winter

More Moisture

The cold winter months call for lots and lots of moisture. Continue using a moisturizing agent on your skin, such as coconut oil, and even up the amount if you live in a particularly cold region. Make sure to treat your whole body to moisture because even with layers on, the cold air will penetrate and affect every bit of skin. Add extra moisture at night to keep skin hydrated and ready to go in the morning.

Vitamin A

Winter is also a good time to increase your application of Vitamin A or retinol. This anti-aging ingredient is great to use to keep the skin in peak condition, but it tends to be photosensitive so using it during months when the sun isn't out as much is best.

You can find retinol, vitamin A, in many products, but a simple way to add in Vitamin A is to use rosehip seed oil. A great source of Vitamin A, this oil can be added to your skincare routine during the winter months. It is best applied at night, to limit its exposure to the sun, and only every other day to let your body get acclimated to it.

Hydration

One thing many people forget during the winter is to stay hydrated. The skin is one of the organs in our bodies that needs the most water to be able to stay in peak condition.

Although during the winter we tend to drink more teas, hot cocoa or other hot drinks, don't forget to keep your intake of water high as well since your skin needs as much moisture as it can get. Applying moisturizer on the outside will only get you so far if you're not staying properly hydrated on the inside.

Combine and Continue

Skincare is a process that takes months to reach its peak and for you to see benefits. Don't get discouraged if your natural skin care regimen doesn't show results immediately.

The skin takes time to adjust to things just like the rest of your body does. Natural skin care is better and less toxic for your skin, even though it might take awhile to take effect. Continue with the skin care ingredients and products that you see are working for your skin type.

Chapter 10 - Starting Your New Skincare Routine

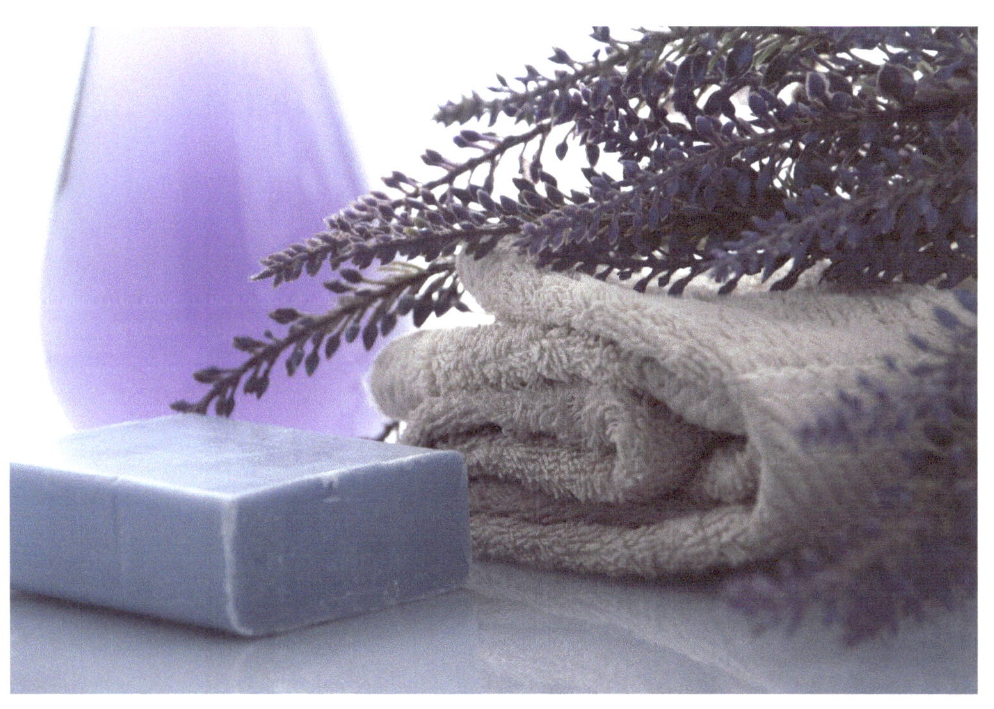

Now that you have all the information you need about going natural with your skincare, you can start developing a routine that works well for you. Remember that not everything has to be 100% natural and homemade, though that is a great way to customize the products going on your skin. Here are some tips for starting a new natural skincare routine:

Go Through Your Current Skincare Products

The first step to starting a new natural skincare routine is to get rid of some of your current products. Don't forget to check the list of toxic ingredients to avoid from Chapter 7. As a refresher, here are some chemical ingredients to beware of:

Parabens
Phthalates
DEA, TEA
PEG Compounds
Propylene Glycol
Petrolatum

Get rid of anything you don't feel comfortable using or that doesn't contain natural and organic ingredients, so you can start fresh.

Consider Your Skin Type and Preferences

Once you have cleaned out your makeup drawer and are ready to start fresh, you will need to think about what you really need for your skin. Consider what your skin type is to start with, such as dry, oily, or combination skin. This can determine what ingredients to look for in your skincare products.

For example, if you have oily skin, you want to be careful with how much oil (even natural oil) is in your products. With dry skin, look for natural oils like coconut or argan oil. You can talk to your dermatologist if you aren't sure what skin type you have.

Another consideration is looking at any skin conditions you have, such as rosacea, eczema, or psoriasis. Certain ingredients don't react well with some types of skin conditions, so be careful with the products you choose.

Test New Products on a Small Area of Skin

When you start using any new skincare products, you should always test new products on a small area of your skin to see how it reacts.

Does it get dry, burn, itch, or turn red? If so, you might be having an allergic reaction, so you should stop using it immediately. Make a list of any products that don't have a good reaction so you can narrow down what ingredients are causing the reaction.

Try Some DIY Skincare Products

There are a lot of amazing store-bought products by natural skincare companies, but you might want to make your own products. There are so many different products you could make, including lotions, cleansers, masks, and serums. Be adventurous and creative! It can be fun and rewarding to make your own products!

Here is a list of natural ingredients that work great in DIY skincare products that you probably already have in your kitchen:

Baking soda
Raw honey
Sugar – white and brown
Salt – pink Himalayan sea salt or regular table salt
Fruit – avocados, bananas, kiwi,

Taking Better Care of Your Skin

Finally, we are convinced you will look and feel more confident when you commit to using natural products on your skin. You don't have to switch to a 100% organic and natural skincare regimen, but the more products you use without harsh and toxic ingredients, the better off your skin will be. It will be healthier, less prone to breakouts, softer, and have a nice, natural glow. Using the tips and tricks of natural skincare in this book will help improve your skin no matter what your goal is, whether it be reducing acne, turning back the clock on aging skin, or simply to protect your skin from harsh chemical ingredients. It's never too late to begin and enjoy the healthier new skin you're in!